WALKING IN AN ANCIENT FOREST

A meditative story to massage your body
and relax your mind

BOOKS IN THE NATUREBODY® SERIES

—

Walking in an Ancient Forest

Camping Under the Night Sky

Relaxing by a Waterfall

A Peaceful Winter Ski

Swimming in a Tropical Sea

A Healing Coastal Walk

Relaxing in the High Desert

A Spirited Mountain Hike

The complete
NatureBody® Connection
program is available at

www.aquaterramassage.com

A NATUREBODY® MASSAGE STORY

Walking in an
ANCIENT
FOREST

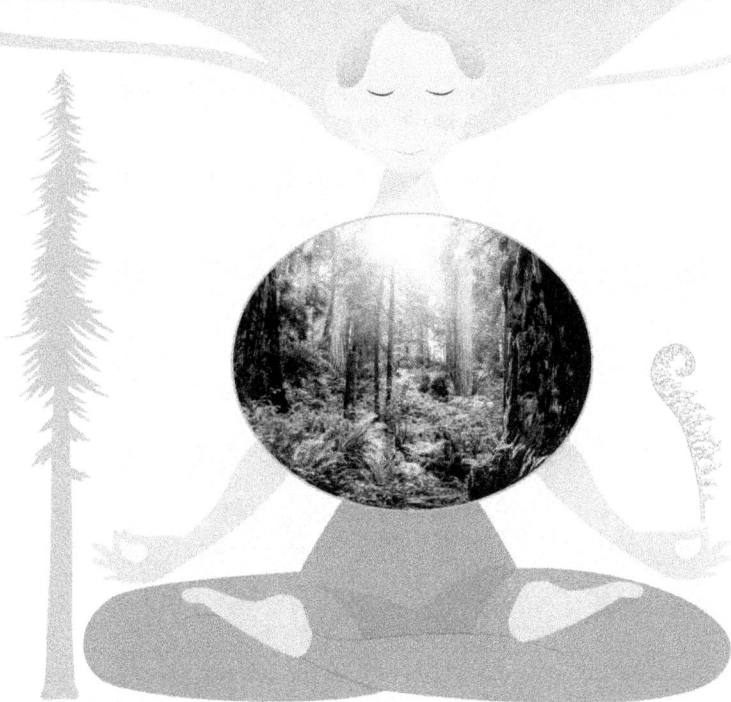

A meditative story to massage your body
and relax your mind

ERIK KRIPPNER *and* FAYE KRIPPNER

Dedicated to you.

*May you find renewed connection
to your incredible body
as you journey across this
magnificent planet.*

Index of Reflections

Contents

A WORD FROM THE AUTHORS

How to Use This Book

Humans have lived in balance with our bodies and the earth for 2.6 million years. Our bodies are designed for this planet. It is natural to walk on uneven ground, climb mountains, run long distances, swim, and most of all, to deeply breathe fresh air. Our wild planet heals and strengthens us by making us more flexible and fluid.

Your body is born of this earth. Earth is here to support you. Unfortunately, the stresses of life pull us off balance, and can leave us feeling physically sore and mentally anxious. This creative journey into relaxation is a way to remember your natural balance and create new muscle memories.

As massage therapists, we understand how a relaxed body feels: how it breathes, how it moves, how it is balanced in space. This NatureBody® massage story shares the full spectrum of massage: body, mind and spirit. Our intention is to empower you to find healing within yourself.

Visualization can have powerful effects on your body.[1] In this guided visualization, you will exercise your mind and imagination to deeply relax and bring your body back to center.

If you are injured or your ability to move is limited, then visualization is even more important! Studies have shown that when you imagine moving, the same areas of your brain activate as if you are actually moving those specific muscles.[2] Through visualization, you are virtually exercising your body.

We are intending for you to have a tangible, physical response to the ideas in this book. The power of this story lies in the vividness of your imagination. Read slowly. Pause. Use all of your senses to experience the story. Imagine the changes in humidity. Feel the gentle breeze on your skin. Hear the soothing sound of the wind. Smell the fresh scent of the life around you. Use your vibrant imagination to experience every detail in this story.

Put yourself in the story. Try to experience every sensation in your body. If you feel like moving, do it! Trust your instincts. Imagine what it feels like to move through the story: your muscles warming and stretching... your breathing deepening... your heartbeat slowing as you deeply relax. Let these sensations come to you at the speed of thought. This isn't about concentrating as much as it is about experiencing.

Each time you practice visualizing this story, your experience will become more vibrant. Your body is your wilderness to explore and understand. Your mind is your canvas for new muscle memories.

The Reflections are our personal notes to you. They offer you insight into some of the concepts in the story. Use them to spark your own creative thoughts about connection and healing.

The Notes section is full of wonderful articles and books that we have selected for you. If you feel interested in a topic, we highly recommend you look at the notes to explore the topic further.

The Journal at the end of the book gives you an opportunity to enhance and deepen your meditation. We have asked you a few thought-provoking questions to help you get started. Feel free to write or draw. Journal as creatively as you are inspired. This is your time to dream of the supportive connections between your body and nature.

There is much to discover about your relationship with your body and the beautiful world around you. Find a comfortable place to relax and enjoy. Prepare to be transported to a setting where you can unwind, immersed in nature, and experience the unbridled freedom of the wild!

From Wellness To Oneness,

Erik and Faye
Your Virtual Massage Therapists

FROM WELLNESS TO ONENESS

Wherever you are,

however you feel,

whatever your state of wellness,

know that

healing is at hand.

Your body is always seeking balance

and looking for opportunities to restore.

Through wellness,

may you come to oneness

with your body,

your mind,

your spirit,

and the beautiful Earth that supports us all.

ABOUT THIS MEDITATION

Introduction

T here is something deeply relaxing about being in a forest. Studies have shown that walking in a forest lowers your blood pressure and heart rate.[3] This NatureBody® meditation guides you on a relaxing walk through an old growth forest.

Let your mind flow into a healing daydream as you imagine yourself strolling through this tranquil wilderness. Imagine wise, giant trees towering above you. Feel the gentle caress of a breeze on your cheek.

The thrum of life penetrates every breath on this earth. Our lives on land are connected to the sea and the air. There is no separation.

We hope that this NatureBody® massage meditation helps you feel more relaxed and connected in the world.

To experience the entire

NatureBody® Connection

scan this QR code

or go to

www.aquaterramassage.com / naturebodygift / ancientforest

A gift for you, dear reader.

A special reading by the authors awaits you
at the link above.

CHAPTER ONE

Welcome

BREATHING AND THORACIC MASSAGE

I stand peacefully in an ancient forest. Moss hangs in the giant trees, and covers the rocks.

> *There is a quiet stillness in this beautiful grove*
> *-a harmonic hush-*
> *the presence of life both seen and unseen.*

Mist hovers in the air. Trees drip its cool, condensed freshness.

Fluffy, green moss and multicolored tapestries of lichens adorn the feet of the trees. Ferns spring up in the spaces between their toes.

Ancient trees stand tall, bearing their wisdom of centuries. Their immense forms soar high to branches far above. A bird glides smoothly from tree to tree, skillfully

Breathing to Relax

"My breath slows, sinking down to my abdomen."

Sometimes the simplest things can feel like magic. Simply breathing has the power to relax you.

Your nervous system controls both voluntary and involuntary actions of your body. Voluntary movements are the things you do consciously, whereas involuntary actions happen even while you sleep.

Breathing is special because it bridges both the conscious and the unconscious parts of our nervous system.

Different patterns of breathing communicate different messages to your unconscious mind. Short, shallow breathing brings you into the fight or flight state, which might be helpful to get energized before an event. Slow, deep breathing brings you into the parasympathetic state, where your body naturally spends its energy on healing and digestion.

Breathing is a subtle yet powerful way to become healthier.

savoring the cornucopia of the canopy.

This peaceful setting invites me to take a few moments to
breathe, to ground, to center. I begin by observing my
breath.

I place my hands on my sides
and feel them widen as I inhale.

I exhale, letting my ribcage narrow.

My breath slows, sinking down to my abdomen.

...I let my breath fill my body.

My torso widens as I inhale.

My shoulders drop with each exhale.

My inhale lengthens my spine,
the spaces between the vertebrae
becoming more dynamic.

...I let my breath fill my body.

As I exhale, I maintain this space, keeping my spine long.

I imagine inhaling into my sacrum.

...I let my breath fill my body.

On my exhale, I retain the openness in my low back.

Calming Body, Mind and Spirit

"I am encouraging my body into the calm, restful state, where I am most receptive to healing."

There are many ways to relax: body, mind, and spirit.

To relax your physical body, find a slow, calm, diaphragmatic breath. Breathe low into your abdomen. Exhale slowly and completely. Emphasize your exhales; let your inhales come naturally.

To relax your mind, focus on positive thoughts that give you a sense of warmth and comfort. Visualization is a powerful tool to communicate to your mind that all is well.[4]

Nurture your spirit by giving. When we give to others, we are rewarded with a feeling of gratitude and abundance. Even giving to your body counts! Stretch your muscles. Drink some water. Go for a walk.

Being in nature is a wonderful way to relax your whole self: body, mind, and spirit. "Forest bathing," or spending mindful time in the outdoors, has been shown to have profound healing effects.[5]

When you are relaxed, your body switches out of the survival mode and into a "rest and digest" mode, where it focuses on your health, well-being and longevity.

I slow my breath, allowing time for my exhale
    to naturally leave my lungs.

...I let my breath fill my body.

My belly expands and contracts as I breathe.

As I draw breath into my low belly,
    I am encouraging my body into the calm, restful state,
    where I am most receptive to healing.

Through breathing,
    I am communicating with my subconscious,
    reassuring it that I am perfectly safe
    in this place,
    in this moment.

...I allow my breath to fill my body.

I am especially aware of the space
    between the exhale and the next inhale.

My breath deepens further,
    filling my hips, all the way down to my legs.

...My breath fills my body.

My breathing has become satisfying and effortless. My tissues continue to open and soften with each breath.

I am present in this moment, in the center of this protected grove: relaxed, warm, and ready to walk.

CHAPTER TWO

Connecting with the Forest

METABOLISM AND SENSORY MASSAGE

I am standing in a shaded grove of an ancient forest. Giant evergreens tower above me. These trees have existed together for centuries. They have witnessed life change as their roots weave a fabric of life, support, and communication beneath the soil.

It is a misty day, and a soft veil of suspended cloud vapor hovers in the air. The grey sky gives the greens of the forest plants a neon glow. Each needle of every tree is outlined with the silver mist.

A trail lies ahead of me. It invites me to follow its meandering path. A cool breeze wraps around me, gently whispering of the delights ahead.

The first step on the trail excites me. I wonder what mysteries await.

The Healing Power of Scent

"I am steeped in the sweet scent of the forest."

Mindfulness is a state of being aware of the sensations you are experiencing, both inside and outside your body.

Noticing scent is a mindful tool to immerse yourself in the moment.

Close your eyes and inhale the scent of the air. Without judgment, accept the aromas that you notice.

You are awakening your brain to the atmosphere around you. By focusing on scent, you are bringing yourself into the present moment: a space of mindfulness and healing.

The scents of the natural world are particularly restorative. The aromas of plants have many healing properties.[6] Cedar and wild rose both have been found to have calming and uplifting effects. Peppermint and pine are energizing.

Whether you take a walk in the forest or enjoy essential oils at home, the scents of nature are wonderful tools for your health.

I walk slowly along the winding path through the ancient forest. The quiet rhythm of my footsteps is soothing. I relax into a meditative pace.

As I look through the forest, I notice ferns of many varieties. Prehistoric sword ferns point proudly to the sky. Their fronds are glossy with dewdrops. Delicate lady ferns gracefully brush the ground with their soft, lacy fronds. Fresh, young fiddleheads unfurl from the tips of newborn shoots.

Even up in the mossy branches of the trees, ferns have found a home, adding to the variety of life in the tree canopy.

I am steeped in the sweet scent of the forest. Cedars and conifers infuse the air with a spicy aromatic evergreen fragrance. The air is lightened with the sweet scent of mountain rose. Contrasting scents blend together in a unique, ambrosial perfume.

As misty dewdrops moisten the soil, the deep, pungent aroma of earth wells up.

I am bathed in the forest's fragrance. It will linger in my awareness long after my walk has finished.

The path makes slight turns, winding between trees and following the contours of the earth. It rises and falls gently and I glide along it, my legs moving easily and freely.

I breathe in.

The air is cool and moist and fresh.

My belly expands with my inhale.

On a Balanced Spine

*"My spine stretches tall as if I were one of
the towering trees, reaching for the sky."*

It takes less muscular effort to hold ourselves upright
when our bones are aligned and our structure is balanced.

Our abdominal muscles support our spine so it can be
strong and flexible. This tall, supported posture releases
other muscles in our bodies. We become more free to
move and flow.

Being off balance leads to a chain reaction of tension
through our bodies. When we don't use our abs to hold
ourselves up, other muscles try to take on the
responsibility. Our low backs and shoulders become tight.
Even our knees and feet respond to the change in balance.

Try this exercise. Stand tall. Keep your weight even
through both of your feet. Support your spine by engaging
your abs. Keep your eyes level, gazing into the distance.

Let your shoulder blades sink down your back. Feel your
neck lengthen and your throat soften. Notice your arms
able to swing more freely. The gentle support from your
core frees your form to be more fluid.

Clean air flows deep into my lower body,
my hips,
my pelvis.

I imagine my body rising as it is filled with the forest air,
floating as if my feet are touching the earth
more tenderly.

As I wander, I imagine my inhales flowing down my legs and through my feet. I feel an energetic connection with the earth beyond the surface to the roots below.

I step more softly,
wanting the soles of my feet to feel more vividly.

My spine stretches tall as if I were one of the towering trees,
reaching for the sky.

My limbs swing freely,
in natural cadence to the energy
rising out of my vital core.

I am at once part of the subterranean world
and the forest canopy.

I imagine my feet reaching down through the earth
while the crown of my head rises to the highest branches.

My presence fills the forest
as I glide smoothly along the path.

I am a part of this landscape.

Moving Beyond Limitations

"This energetic awareness opens my being..."

Close your eyes. Feel the atmosphere around you. Feel the air on your skin.

Smell the aromas drifting in the air. Listen to the sounds around you. Notice your feet on the earth.

Feel the vibration of all that is around you. Your body and mind resonate with the outer world.

Having a sense of your deep connection with Mother Earth can empower you to move more fluidly, to fire your muscles more powerfully, to breathe with true inspiration.

Visualize yourself as an energetic being with unlimited potential for flow, for healing, and for change.

Each breath grounds me.

I am buoyed and supported by the forest.

My being is enlightened: powerful with this new energy. I am more aware of that which surrounds me, and that which is within me. This energetic awareness opens my being to the harmonies of energy that compose this forest song.

The song of the forest beckons.

I walk to answer its call.

I breathe to join its song.

Walk on, Tranquil Wanderer.

CHAPTER THREE

The Communicative Earth

FEET AND NERVOUS SYSTEM

I am light of foot, balanced and centered as I meander along the winding trail.

The forest soil is alive. Plant and animal life tunnel through the nutrients of planet Earth for nourishment and structure.

Vast networks of fungal filaments, like galaxies throughout the soil, offer food and communication, essential to life itself. Fungi conduct the chemical communication for all plants. Through their network, trees translate nutrients into nourishment and communicate with one another.

The path gently descends. The trees are widely spaced and a carpet of purple flowers covers the forest floor. This high mountain forest is moist from lingering snows and extra rain afforded by its elevated perch.

On Bare Feet

*"My feet are pliable and flexible. With each step,
they contour to the earth."*

Faye and I spent a summer walking 1200 miles on the
Appalachian Trail from Georgia to Pennsylvania in
barefoot shoes. These flexible shoes gave us the minimalist
protection of a moccasin. They allowed our feet to move
freely while protecting us from sharp rocks and sticks. We
enjoyed the freedom of movement and the stable balance
of walking barefoot.

Walking barefoot allows our toes to spread wide,
providing a stable foundation. Skin, fat, and muscle tissue
cushion our feet in just the right places. The arches of our
feet absorb powerful forces, allowing the small bones of
our feet to support our entire structure.

Our feet are designed to conform to the natural ground.
To feel with our feet is to awaken their elegant, dynamic
strength. The soles of our feet have thousands of nerve
endings. They are in constant conversation with their
environment.

Walking barefoot can strengthen your feet and improve
your balance.

Even a few water-loving cottonwoods and big leaf maple trees have found a home here. Small squirrels run up and down their trunks, chattering at one another.

> *I brush my foot across the trail, lightly sensing*
> *the moisture of the earth and the scattered fir needles*
> *contrasted against the dark, rich soil.*

> *I detect the vibration of the living earth, life flowing just*
> *below the superficial crust of the path.*

> *My feet are pliable and flexible.*

> *With each step, they contour to the earth.*

> *The bones of my feet spread wide across the ground.*

> *The beautiful arch of the foot, made of tiny bones,*
> *carries the weight of my whole body.*

But, my feet were created for more than carrying the weight of my world. With thousands of nerve endings, they were designed to read the terrain upon which I walk.

They detect details of each step I take: the "personality" of the earth.

Walking tall and light, I instinctively adjust my stride to harmonize with the contours beneath my feet. The topography challenges my feet to become stronger, more supple, as they move across the natural landscape.

> *I imagine an energetic connection with the earth,*
> *stepping softly to feel more vividly.*

On Fungi

*"Just beneath the surface of the soil,
the fungal web detects my presence."*

Mushrooms are the small fruiting bodies of a vastly complex organism.

Under every mushroom, just below the surface of the soil, an extensive network of filaments branches out, joining with other fungi to form a mycelial web. This web connects the roots of trees and all life.

Trees use this mycelial web to nourish themselves and each other, as well as to communicate with the rest of the forest. When a tree is distressed, other trees nearby will feed and support it using the mycelial web.

Imagine fungi as the nervous system of the forest.

As you walk, picture the living earth vibrating with the electrical current of the mycelial web, pulsing with communication. Rather than thudding your feet on lifeless ground, let your feet spring lightly upon the living soil. Allow the soles your feet to listen to the earth.

Walking with a strong yet supple, receptive stride can help your whole body move more smoothly.

My walk becomes a dance with the dynamic ground.

The path winds through an inviting blanket
of fresh, spring-green wood sorrel.

It crushes its cool, green aroma under my feet.

The maple tree's renewing form
scatters textures of twigs along my golden-leafed path.

Sinewy roots emerge out of the ground.

My feet spread and conform to the curves.

Each step is individual, unique.

The texture of the path builds character in my tissues.

The muscles of my feet know how to work, how to press into the earth and launch me forward into my next step. I appreciate each step, even the uncomfortable ones. My feet keep me aware and present in this moment.

I pause. Just beneath the surface of the soil, the fungal web detects my presence. On some level, my feet must also detect this communication singing through the soil.

The high mountain forest ends at a mountain bluff. The trail leads through the rocky fortress, descending to a forested valley below. I pause to look back up at the terrain I have just covered, and drink in the perspective that my two legs have brought me.

CHAPTER FOUR

Walking by the Silvery Stream

LEGS, HIPS, AND CIRCULATION

A s the trail descends into the forested valley, a mosaic of life opens before me. Rhododendrons and azaleas add color to the forest tapestry.

I feel the locomotion of my hips, knees, and ankles.
My legs become more active and nimble.

Some steps, I lean heavily on my legs.
Others are as light as wisp of breeze on a mirror lake.

A silvery stream slips between the trees. Round, gray rocks line the edges of the stream. Stepping stones protrude from the shallows.

The presence of water is delightful.

A New Pattern of Movement

"My body is challenged in new ways..."

Our bodies are constantly adapting to our demands. The muscles we use get stronger. The muscles we stretch become more flexible. The muscles we don't use atrophy.

Challenging your muscles to fire in new ways can restore balance to your body. When you try new activities and move in different ways, many positive changes occur. Weak muscles become stronger. Tight muscles begin to stretch. New neural pathways are established in your brain. Circulation flows to restore stagnant tissues.

Nature can inspire us to move in new ways. From running like the wind or prowling like a cat, to simply walking on uneven terrain, our bodies are constantly challenged, strengthened and recharged in the natural world.

As the valley dips, the stream stair-steps downward in little waterfalls. Water rushes around the stones, giving the stream a voice. It babbles and chatters as it ripples down the rapids. The fresh, clean smell of ozone emanates from the rambling brook.

This valley is full and abundant. Life abounds from the highest points of the canopy, where birds alight in the tops of the trees, down to the most delicate succulents next to the stream bed below. The profile of life feels whole in this abundant, protected valley. The valley is alive.

The stream follows the folds of the hills, winding back and forth across the trail. The path has more curves and dips in it now. It disappears into the stream and emerges on the opposite bank. I step lightly from rock to rock as I cross the stream.

The trail is fun to walk, with its many small rises and bends. I am pleasantly focused, looking for the next place to step.

A tree has fallen across the trail. I take a giant step over it. These longer, wider steps are deeply satisfying.

My body is challenged in new ways, and I feel the rush of circulation thrumming through me.

Walking across this pleasant landscape,
my legs begin to feel stronger
-springier-
and my joints ease.

Movement and stretching feel natural.

My knees become more fluid and flexible.

On Squatting

*"I bend deeper into a squat. My spine lengthens
as the spaces between my vertebrae open."*

For millennia, humans' natural resting position has been a
deep squat. Young children naturally squat as they play. In
many cultures, squatting is still a natural way of resting
for all people, young and old.[7]

Our bodies are not well adapted to sitting on chairs.
Sitting can cause our spinal discs to compress.

Squatting, being our natural way of resting, has many
physical benefits.[8] When you squat, your weight is evenly
balanced between the muscles of your legs, hips, and core.
Your spine decompresses. Your achilles tendons stretch. A
deep squat stimulates your digestion.

To get your body accustomed to a deep squat, start by
lying down and hugging your knees into your chest. Circle
your legs with your hands on your knees to lubricate your
hip joints and free your pelvis and low back.

Next, from a standing position, try lowering yourself into
a squat, slowly and shallowly at first, with your feet wide
apart. Keep the movement comfortable. It is better to take
many tries, bending a little deeper each time, than do too
much at once. Be patient with your body. Even small,
consistent changes can make a big difference.

I am able to bend deeply and comfortably.

I kneel down to look more closely at the moss lining the stream. What was just a patch of green, now is revealed to be a bejeweled world. Shimmering droplets, lightly balanced on the moss, add a silvery radiance. Tiny, feathery green leaflets wave gently back and forth in the wind of moving water.

A minnow maneuvers upstream, darting under the moss for protection.

I bend deeper into a squat.

My spine lengthens as the spaces between my vertebrae open.

I feel the last remaining tension in my back easing.

I inhale.

Breath enters deep into my pelvis,
as if my sitz bones are adjusting to make more space.

I push through my heels to stand, pleased to feel my strong and resilient legs under me.

I am thankful for this wonderful walk and to be a part of Mother Nature's brilliant design.

CHAPTER FIVE

The Sounds of the Forest

HEAD MASSAGE

T he trail continues down the valley. It meanders away from the stream up to a quiet stand of giant fir trees. There is less undergrowth now: the forest is shading the ground.

I look at the trees around me: huge Goliaths, evenly spaced. I reach around a tree to see how big it is. My outstretched arms don't begin to measure. I feel humbled to be in this sacred grove, among wise giants.

I am standing near a grand fir. I follow its gray furrowed trunk with my eyes up to its silvery smooth branches. It is over a hundred feet tall, and yet I can still see the fir needles clearly. They create a herringbone pattern, silhouetted against the white, white sky. Each tree reaches its branches toward its neighbor, filtering the gray-washed day into dappled green light, in this natural cathedral.

On Listening

*"These trees have stories to tell me,
if I could only listen sensitively enough."*

One ear of an owl is higher than the other. That placement allows them to tell if a sound is coming not only from the left or the right, but also from above or below.[9] They have spatial awareness of their environment through sound.

Close your eyes and listen to the world around you. What do you hear? Now listen more deeply, to the quiet beneath those first sounds. Turn and tilt your head to detect and locate the soundscape around you.

As you reach to listen to ever quieter sounds, notice the sensations in your head. Feel your jaw relax. Feel the temporal bones on the sides of your skull adjust as your ears reach to hear. Notice your neck lengthening and your throat softening. Let your head swivel on your spine as you turn it from side to side.

Turn your focus within. Become still and listen softly enough to hear your own internal self. At this level, listening blends with feeling. If you cover your ears, you can still hear the beating of your heart. You are listening with your whole body, not just your ears.

The act of listening is a sensitive tool to connect to the world around and within you.

Standing in the quiet of the old growth forest,
    I marvel at the depth of silence.

The trees seem to soak in sound,
    absorbing stress, worry, and anxiety;
    resonating peace,
    silence,
    and timelessness.

Majestic firs, hemlocks and cedars born in a long-past
era stand tall, individually strong, and intricately connected
through their root systems. I imagine their roots plunging
deep into the soil, as deep as the trees are tall, and nearly
twice as wide.

Delicate strands of mycelium envelop the roots in a silken
shroud, bringing the nourishment of the earth to animate
the life of the tree. This intricate web of roots binds the soil
together. I feel held and supported by Mother Nature's
ancient wisdom.

These trees have stories to tell me,
    if I could only listen sensitively enough.

I try, holding still for a few moments.

I close my eyes and soften my face,
    my jaw,
    my neck,
    allowing my awareness and presence
    to wash into my ears.

On Silence

*"My ears open as I draw in faint and subtle sounds
from the forest around me."*

We are surrounded by human-produced noise. Even on a
quiet day, you might notice the hum of a fan, distant
airplanes, the quiet whirr of the refrigerator, or the
murmur of conversation in another room. Our human
world is enveloped in these various vibrations.

In the quiet of a forest, the natural soundscape produces a
silence alive with the sounds of nature. Water drips on
leaves. A distant frog croaks. Birds rustle through the
leaves. A breeze whispers through the forest.

All of these sounds compose nature's symphony. They
stimulate our auditory complex in a relaxing way.[10] Listen
closely to the sounds around you and notice the sensations
in your ears and jaw.

The unpredictable nature of a living soundscape heightens
our senses to the world around us.

Even quiet places can be alive with sound.

There is a silence, a deep stillness
  that draws me into the power,
  the wisdom,
  and the peace of this moment.

I feel connected to a timelessness that permeates the forest.

My awareness softens
  and the deep stillness begins to speak.

My ears open as I draw in faint and subtle sounds
  from the forest around me.

I hear the rustling of a leaf as a raindrop rolls down its glossy surface and off its tip. Birds stir softly in the rhododendrons. In the distance, a woodpecker taps against a Douglas-fir tree.

A faint tendril of breeze whispers toward me. I follow its swirling path through the trees, swelling as it makes its way closer, until it is above me. I sense its presence, stirring the air around me. I look up. The branches above me wave gently as if welcoming the breeze. Its jovial, spirit-like presence diminishes as it continues on its journey through the treetops, until it is a distant hush...and then...silence returns.

My breathing feels refreshed with the passing breeze, the
  fresh, clean mountain air flushing through my being.

This energetic awareness opens my being to the harmonies of
  energy that compose this forest song.

The song of the forest beckons. Hike on, Tranquil Wanderer.

CHAPTER SIX

The Shapes of Nature

RELAXING EYES AND SINUSES

I walk past large Douglas-fir trees, admiring the thick bark, known as phloem, that insulates and protects them. Thickly braided ridges in the bark travel up the tree to a spiral of branches completing a triangular treetop.

Wherever I look in the forest, I see designs. Mother Nature's designs extend far beyond simple geometry: squares, triangles, spheres. The patterns of nature are vastly more complex. The forest is made up of a series of repeating patterns called "fractals." The complexity of forest patterns brings peace to my brain.

A single tree rises out of the ground. Large branches extend from its trunk, splitting into smaller and smaller branches and twigs. And twigs yet further into needles. A singular form branching repeatedly into smaller and smaller forms that resemble the original.

The Patterns of Nature

"Everywhere I look, I see these repeating patterns."

Euclid is the father of geometry. He studied simple, smooth shapes: squares, triangles, and circles. In our cities, it is easy to see Euclid's influence all around us: we are in a world of geometric shapes.[11]

When we are in nature, we see a different world, rough and textured. All around us are shapes with jagged edges and branching patterns. From braided rivers to the veins of leaves, the rugged edges of a mountain to the jagged profile of a coastline seen from above, nature is designed with fractal geometry.

Fractal design is a complex branching, repeating form: a never-ending pattern that is repeated from large to small, to smaller and ever smaller.[12]

Your body is an elegant design, and as beautifully complex as nature intended. Fractals are part of your anatomy.[13] Your lungs, your venous system, the sound of your heartbeat, the neural patterns of your mind, are all fractal forms.

You belong in nature. You are one of its perfect forms. Your body shares immeasurable beauty, inside and out.

You are part of nature's perfection.

Everywhere I look, I see these repeating patterns. The curled stalk of a young fern holds curled fronds, like fingers. When I look closely at these fronds, I see tiny leaflets, nestled in little curls within each frond.

These intricate patterns create the textures of nature, like the concentric rings of lichen, patiently digesting mountains, to the soft seeds of a dandelion, carrying the wishes of future. A dandelion wish, or capitulum, is a sphere of soft projections, that in turn split into little wings, ready to be blown by the wind and set sail. Their fuzziness is a gift of fractal design.

Fractal design is in my structure as well. As I breathe, the air enters my trachea, which divides into bronchi, which continually divide into ever smaller bronchioles, creating a vast network of air passages in my lungs. At the ends of the bronchioles, tiny alveoli, or air sacs, translate the atmosphere to my bloodstream.

> *Like inverted trees, my lungs exchange*
> *the gas of the atmosphere with that of my bloodstream.*

> *With each exhale, I give the plants around me the*
> *sustenance they need.*

> *With each inhale, I take in their exhaled oxygen.*

> *Flora and fauna exist as yin and yang,*
> *nourishing each other naturally.*

> *The forest and I belong together.*

Mind Massage

*"My brain is excited, yet soothed, by the patterns
that my eyes are born to see."*

Fractals are complex shapes, and yet our brains relax when
we see them. We have been surrounded by the fractal
designs in nature since the dawn of humanity. As we gaze
at fractal patterns, our minds become pleasantly occupied.
This helps us to be aware without focusing. We drift into
mindfulness.

Studies have found that looking at fractals in nature
increases alpha brainwave activity.[4] Alpha waves occur in
the brain when we are relaxed, meditating, or
daydreaming. Simply looking at fractals is relaxing.

A walk in nature is like moving through a living
kaleidoscope, abundant with the complex patterns of
nature. Allow your mind to dance from the analytical to
the artistic. Letting your mind relax as your eyes drink in
the scenery around you, you are beginning to see the forest
for the trees.

Go beyond *looking* and *see*.

Each glance into the trees draws me into a deeper focus. Patterns repeat from large to small, small to large. My eyes enjoy deciphering in ever more detail, these intricate visual harmonies.

As if visually feasting upon the fractal nature of the woodland plants, the more I look at something the more I notice. My brain is excited, yet soothed, by the patterns that my eyes are born to see.

I pick up a pinecone that has dropped to the forest floor. When I turn it upside down, I see dual-spiral patterns, winding their way in opposite directions formed by the diamonds of each apophysis and the pointy umbo in the center of each. I am impressed that a pinecone can look so reminiscent of the center of a sunflower in full bloom.[5]

My gaze is relaxed as I look into the forest.

My body is warm and flowing.

A feeling of oneness fills my spirit and sends me down the trail at a lively clip.

Walk on, Tranquil Wanderer.

CHAPTER SEVEN

Communing with the Forest

A FULL BODY RELAXATION

I continue walking along the forest valley. Time feels irrelevant. I am here...now...in this moment. Each step, like a dependable metronome, sounds the cadence of my meditation.

> I wander, enjoying the clean air,
>> the soft ground,
>> the majestic trees towering above.

> I am becoming a closer part of these woods
>> as I deepen my soft focus.

The trail descends down a small hill. Ahead of me, the trees open into a vibrant forest glade. Tufts of elk sedge and beargrass carpet the glade floor, while willows and dogwoods edge this tapestry. I walk across the springy

On Walking Downhill

"The trail descends down a small hill."

Many hikers say that walking downhill is harder than walking uphill. It is easy to relax and let gravity pull us down the hill. When we relax our muscles, the impact of walking puts stress on our joints, especially our knees.

Our muscles act like natural shock absorbers. Activating our leg muscles protects our joints.

When you walk downhill, it is important to visualize your strong, supple, buoyant thigh and calf muscles cushioning impact, easing the pressure of gravity on your joints.

Keep your knees unlocked as you make your way downhill. Let your springy legs adjust to the terrain. Reach strongly for your next step, and pull the earth under you by using your hamstrings.

Keeping your legs strong and active will cushion the impact on your knees, so you can enjoy many more miles in the years to come.

ground, abundant with life. In spring, this meadow is a shallow pond, but the mountain meltwater has passed and the soil is soft and dry.

A small ridge defines the far edge of the glade. This is the last ridge before before these mountains spill out to the open plains beyond. I continue across the glade to where this ridge meets the silvery stream that bisects its mountainous constraints on its way to distant seas.

The lower edge of the glade yields a mountain spring. This lush wet area, encircled by stately trees, brings aquatic life to this quiet forest garden. Large blooms, perfectly adapted to the abundant moisture, lighten the deep shade with sunshine yellow.

As the seep falls gently down to join the main flow, the trees close in to escort the silvery stream through its mountain pass. In its dark, humid shade, I feel a sense of deepening ease, a reverence for my feeling of home and security, here in the mountains.

Pillows of moss irresistibly cover the ground.

I brush my bare feet across the moss.

It is cool and comforting,
and I am ready to rest.

I sit down and then lie back.

The soft moss cushions my body.

The chill from the moist earth
yields quickly to the heat of my body
as it warms the ground underneath me.

Our Need for Water

*"The chill from the moist earth yields
quickly to the heat of my body."*

Moisture transforms a forest. In the dewy morning, during an afternoon rain shower, or on a cloudy day, moisture awakens life in the forest.

When moss dampens, its texture changes from dry and brittle to soft and pillowy. The soil expands with moisture and new life begins to sprout. Water washes leaves, re-exposing their chlorophyll for photosynthesis.

Our bodies also need water to thrive.

We are made of 60 percent water.[16] Our organs, muscles, brain and blood all need water to function.

Even our bones, which seem to be brittle and dry, are actually flexible.[17] Living bone can bend slightly. The inner core of bone, spongy bone, resembles moss with its lattice-like structure.

When we are hydrated and healthy, the water in our bodies helps us to be stronger, increases our energy, aids in digestion and boosts our immunity. Being hydrated even softens our skin, like the moss of the forest.

Water is the elixir of life. Cheers!

I breathe the scent of the forest,
    the dewy moss,
    the bite of evergreen,
    the mushroomy soil,
    and the fresh alpine air.

As I inhale, I feel my ribs expand across the soft ground.

I exhale, and a peaceful heaviness envelops my body.

I allow gravity to work deeply on my entire body.

My toes soften and become limp.

The arches of my feet unwind
    and my heels rest into the moss.

My calves release
    and my knees open gently across the earth.

The relaxation continues up my legs.

My thighs melt into the earth,
    allowing my hips to expand and soften.

Tension in my lower back dissolves,
    and as I breathe, I feel my spine lengthening.

My belly is soft. It rises and falls gently with my breathing.

My ribs sink into the ground and my chest widens,
    allowing my shoulders to melt back into the moss.

On Relaxation

"My body softens into a serene countenance, my whole persona open to the molding of this peaceful energy."

Relaxation can feel elusive. You cannot force yourself to relax. It comes quietly when invited.

A great way to develop your ability to relax is by paying attention to your breathing.

Feel your body breathe.

Notice the sensations in your body. Allow your limbs to become heavy. Let the weight of your body sink while your spine remains long.

Exhale completely. Let your next inhale come slowly and quietly.

These are cues to help you command a conscious, relaxing breath.

Be patient as you develop your calm nature through breath. Let go of your expectations and welcome the feelings that arise.

Be thankful for progress. Relaxation is a breath away.

My arms feel limp and my palms connect softly
    with the earth.

My body is completely relaxed.

My throat softens.
    My neck lengthens.
    My energy feels complete.

I feel long from the center of my arches
    to the crown of my head.

My head sinks back into the supportive moss.

My teeth open and my jaw slackens.
    It feels like my jaw is sinking back into my ears.

My face eases its expressions.
    My eyebrows open,
    my scalp relaxes,
    and my hair cascades back into the moss.

My body softens into a serene countenance,
    my whole persona open to the molding
    of this peaceful energy.

I rest into the moss, the earth, the root systems of the ancient
    trees. I have blended into this eternal timelessness.

My consciousness is free, experiencing the dreams of the forest.

CHAPTER EIGHT

Gratitude

A BLESSING FROM THE ELEMENTS

T hank you for joining me on this hike today. Many great thinkers spend hours in quiet contemplation, deeply immersed in the enjoyment and wonder that we have experienced here together. May your body feel refreshed and renewed through this dance of mind. Until we meet again,

> *May Earth nourish you.*
>
> *May air elevate your spirit.*
>
> *May water teach your love to flow.*
>
> *May the fires of life warm your soul,*
>   *that others may bask in its radiance.*

Dream on, Tranquil Wanderer.

Acknowledgments

This book is born from a lifelong love of nature, and three decades of study in the natural sciences and the human body.

As with all meaningful achievements, there are many people who have helped to make this possible.

Thank you, first, to our families, who introduced us to the outdoors as young children. The vivid imagination of a child dreams on in us with every outdoor adventure.

A special thanks to Barbara Bollinger: dedicated editor, voiceover coach, cheerleader, advisor and mother. We are sincerely grateful for your presence in our lives. Your vibrant energy radiates throughout this book.

Jane Goodall has inspired us with her message of hope. We can all be a force for healing on this planet.

Thank you to Dr. Robert Noble for guiding Erik to recognize the details of the forest. Thank you to Dr. Frank Anderson for showing Faye the infinite beauty of fractals.

Many thanks to David Suzuki and Wayne Grady for your book, *Tree: A Life Story*. Your beautiful writing inspired us to see the forest *and* the tree as a constant cycle that contains both the one and the many.

Paul Stamets and Louie Schwartzberg brought the mycelial world to life in their film, *Fantastic Fungi*. The gorgeous cinematography and heartfelt stories of the film sparked much of the writing in this book.

We are grateful to TJ Ford for giving us an enthusiastic introduction to human anatomy. Your sensitive touch still inspires us.

Til Luchau's *Advanced Myofascial Techniques* workshop brought visualization to life by having the class evolve from amoeba to human: a beautiful demonstration on the complexity of our human ability to stand on two legs.

Thank you, Teresa Lee, Matt Lueders, Fanina Padykula, and Jessica Talisman for demonstrating elegance of movement in your pilates and gyrotonic lessons.

And lastly, to our massage clients. We treasure the time we spend with you. Thank you for your trust and your honesty. We are forever grateful to you for teaching us so much about the human form.

Notes

1. "What is Imagery?" *Johns Hopkins Medicine*, 2003, www.hopkinsmedicine.org/health/wellness-and-prevention/imagery.

2. Lohr, Jim. "Can Visualizing Your Body Doing Something Help You Learn to Do It Better?" *Scientific American*, 1 May 2015, www.scientificamerican.com/article/can-visualizing-your-body-doing-something-help-you-learn-to-do-it-better.

3. Park, Bum Jin et al. "The Physiological Effects of Shinrin-yoku (Taking In the Forest Atmosphere or Forest Bathing): evidence from field experiments in 24 forests across Japan." *Environmental Health and Preventive Medicine* vol. 15 no. 1, 2010, pp. 18-26. doi:10.1007/s12199-009-0086-9.

4. Malz, Maxwell. *Psycho-Cybernetics: Updated and Expanded.* New York, NY: Perigee, 2015.

5. Li, Dr. Qing. *Forest Bathing: How Trees Can Help You Find Health and Happiness*. New York, NY: Viking, 2018.

6. Worwood, Valerie Ann. *The Complete Book of Essential Oils & Aromatherapy*. San Rafael, CA: New World Library, 1991.

7. Gersema, Emily. "Squatting and Kneeling May Be Better for Your Health Than Sitting." *USC News*, 9 March 2020, news.usc.edu/166572/squatting-kneeling-health-sitting-usc-research.

8. Medaris Miller, Anna. "Forget Sitting Versus Standing. The Real Question Is Should You Squat More?" *US News and World Report*, 12 April 2018, health.usnews.com/wellness/articles/2018-04-12/forget-sitting-versus-standing-the-real-question-is-should-you-squat-more.

9. Lewis, Deane. "Owl Ears and Hearing." *The Owl Pages*, 23 January 2021, www.owlpages.com/owls/articles.php?a=6.

10. Hartwell, Charles. "Researchers Reveal How Sounds of Nature Relax the Brain." *Study Finds*, 6 April 2017, studyfinds.org/nature-sounds-relaxation-stress.

11. "Geometry in Architecture." *Archisoup*, www.archisoup.com/studio-guide/geometry-in-architecture. Accessed 24 February 2023.

12. Li, M., Sterling, L., Khim, J., Kau, A. "Fractals." *Brilliant Worldwide*, brilliant.org/wiki/fractals. Accessed 25 February 2023.

13. Abdul-Aziz, Shamsu. "Symmetry and Fractals in the Lungs." *Yale National Initiative*, teachers.yale.edu/curriculum/viewer/initiative_11.07.01_u. Accessed 23 February 2023.

14. Hagerhall, C M et al. "Human Physiological Benefits of Viewing Nature: EEG Responses To Exact and Statistical Fractal Patterns." *Nonlinear Dynamics, Psychology, and Life Sciences* vol. 19, no. 1, 2015, pp. 1-12, pubmed.ncbi.nlm.nih.gov/25575556/.

15. Leary, Catie. "How the Golden Ratio Manifests in Nature." *Treehugger,* 3 December 2019, www.treehugger.com/how-golden-ratio-manifests-nature-4869736.

16. Sissons, Claire. "What is the average percentage of water in the human body?" *Medical News Today,* 27 May 2020, www.medicalnewstoday.com/articles/what-percentage-of-the-human-body-is-water.

17. Heaney, Robert Proulx and Whedon, G. Donald. "Bone." *Encyclopedia Britannica,* 15 Feb. 2023, www.britannica.com/science/bone-anatomy. Accessed 25 February 2023.

NOTES

MEDITATION

Journal

This journal gives you a place to reflect on your experience as you read and meditate. With every meditation, your library of personal affirmations can grow. Here are some thoughts you might want to record in words or drawings:

What were your favorite phrases in the story?

What physical sensations or changes did you notice in your body before, during and after the meditation?

Reflect on your body. What memories come to mind? What are your healing intentions for the future?

Describe the forest YOU see in this story, using all your senses.

Enjoy dreaming of your body in nature, and exploring the nature of your body.

May

EARTH

nourish you.

"THESE TREES HAVE STORIES TO
TELL ME, IF I COULD ONLY
LISTEN DEEPLY ENOUGH."

MEDITATION

Watch a tree through the autumn season. Its winding, twisting form is revealed as each leaf falls. This tree has lived through floods and droughts. It has felt strong winds on its branches, and spiraled its roots through the earth. It has stayed strong and tall through seasons of growth. Its twisted, knotty structure tells the story of its life.

Your body also has a story to tell. It has held you through your life's storms. It has stood tall through adversity, and adapted and strengthened to the challenges it has been given.

What storms have you weathered? What lessons have you been gifted?

Listening to your body's story is the first step in appreciating its resilience, its strength, and its incredible, unique beauty. Looking within allows you to turn your focus outward, and be in conversation with the world around you: engaging in the relationships of life.

~

"I AM BECOMING A CLOSER PART
OF THESE WOODS AS I DEEPEN
MY SOFT FOCUS."

MEDITATION

When you soften your gaze, you become more aware of all that is around you. Instead of focusing on a particular object, your peripheral vision soaks in the entire scene. You become aware of the life around you, and can see yourself as part of that life. Softening your focus allows you to feel your connection to the world around you.

~

May

AIR

elevate your spirit.

"I FEEL HELD AND SUPPORTED BY
MOTHER NATURE'S ANCIENT
WISDOM."

MEDITATION

Since the dawn of humanity, people have lived in close relationship with nature. Throughout the natural world, species depend on each other for communication and support. When a tree is distressed, other trees support and nourish it through a web of fungal mycelium running through the soil. There are symbiotic relationships between many wild species.

Even if you live in the city, you are intimately connected to the natural world. Your roots extend back before cities, before traffic, before deadlines. You belong to the ancient world, where you are held and supported by a vast network of life. A network that also depends on you.

~

May

WATER

teach your love to flow.

"I AM ENCOURAGING MY BODY INTO THE CALM, RESTFUL STATE, WHERE I AM MOST RECEPTIVE TO HEALING."

MEDITATION

Breathing is the way we communicate with our subconscious bodies. When you slow and soften your breath, you are telling your body that it is safe: that it can ease into relaxation.

When your body is relaxed, it pours its energy into digestion and healing, to keep you healthy and long-lived.

~

"THE BRANCHES ABOVE ME WAVE
GENTLY, AS IF WELCOMING THE
BREEZE."

MEDITATION

The shifting winds: the winds of change. What breezes are coming into your life? New people and opportunities are like breezes, constantly caressing the tree of your life. How do you welcome them?

~

May the

FIRES OF LIFE

warm your soul,

that others

may bask

in its radiance.

"I WALK ACROSS THE SPRINGY
GROUND, ABUNDANT WITH LIFE."

MEDITATION

Look down at the wild earth. Notice the plants and twigs, the fallen leaves and new shoots of growth. Now, begin to look more closely. Notice the fir needles. Watch for the movement of tiny ants and bugs. You might notice miniature flowers, with infinitesimal details. Earth is abundant with life of every size.

~

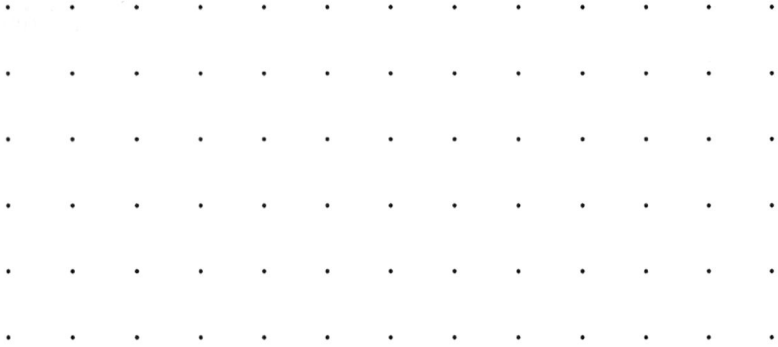

"CONTRASTING SCENTS BLEND
TOGETHER IN A UNIQUE,
AMBROSIAL PERFUME."

MEDITATION

Inhale. Notice the temperature of the air as it enters your nose. Draw the air into your lungs. Feel it spiral in your sinuses. Can you detect the subtle scents riding on tendrils of air?

Exhale. The oxygen and carbon that were once deep in your lungs and your bloodstream are now mingling with the outside air.

As you breathe, feel the exchange of air, like wisps of energy swirling together in the dance of life.

~

BLESSING
OF THE ELEMENTS

May
EARTH
nourish you.

May
AIR
elevate your spirit.

May
WATER
teach your love to flow.

May the
FIRES OF LIFE
warm your soul,
that others
may bask in its radiance.

About the Authors

Born and raised in New Orleans, Erik Krippner grew up with a po'boy in his hand and a song in his heart. As a boy, he spent his summers swimming, hiking, fishing, and sailing. After becoming an Eagle Scout, Erik dreamed of answering the call to "Go West, young man." He earned a Bachelor of Science degree in Forestry from Louisiana State University. Following his passion for adventure, Erik found his way to the mountains of the Pacific Northwest, his home to this day. After working in the forests of Oregon, Washington, Idaho, Alaska, Georgia, and Louisiana, Erik decided to focus his love of natural sciences on the study of human body through massage therapy.

Faye grew up in Oregon surrounded by family and old growth coastal forests. She spent many childhood weekends cross-country skiing, hunting for mushrooms, exploring coastal tide pools, and searching for crawdads in the Siuslaw River. Her love of books deepened when she became the editor of her high school and college's literary journals. Upon earning her Bachelor of Arts degree in Mathematics with honors from the Robert D. Clark Honors College at the University of Oregon, Faye became a technical writer and web developer. The whisper of a deeper purpose ignited her to study massage, where she met Erik.

Erik and Faye became friends in massage school at the East West College of the Healing Arts, in Portland, Oregon. In 2003, they founded Aqua Terra Massage, a therapeutic massage studio for friends and couples. Since then, they have practiced therapeutic massage together, side by side. They have spent years immersed in the study of massage, serving thousands of clients.

Faye and Erik have spent years exploring and writing about our beautiful world. They have sailed the blue waters of Fiji's Koro Sea, kayaked New Zealand's Marlborough Sound, and stargazed among the giraffes and elephants in Botswana. They have hiked the Appalachian Trail and paddled the tidally-influenced Columbia River in the Pacific Northwest. They have seen orca whales swim right under their kayaks, locked eyes with wild lions, and played hide-and-seek with an octopus. They have hiked thousands of miles together, kayaked and sailed hundreds, and spent countless evenings camping under the stars.

With a commitment to bringing more love and kindness to this beautiful world, we offer this book to you.

www.aquaterramassage.com